Live well.

Essential Oils for Wellness, Purpose, and Abundance

Jen O'Sullivan

what are essential oils?

Essential oils are the life-force of plants. They help the plant to regulate itself and add health and overall wellness. These oils can work in much the same way for us. There are three ways to use essential oils: aromatically, topically, and internally. It takes 20 minutes for an essential oil to reach every cell in your body from the time you apply them. There are around 100 trillion cells in our bodies, and one drop of essential oil contains over 40 million trillion molecules! This means every single cell in our body, in 20 minutes, is covered by 400,000 essential oil molecules.

how do you use them?

You may use essential oils in one of three ways: aromatically, topically, and even internally. Each bottle is labeled for proper use. The following are some guidelines to help get you started in the right direction.

AROMATIC: Smell the essential oil directly from the bottle, drip a drop in your palm and cup your hand over your nose to breathe deeply, or use a cold water diffuser with several drops of your favorite oil.

TOPICAL: Place a drop into your palm and rub the essential oil on the back of the neck, bottom of the feet, wrists, spine, top of the head, or anywhere there is a need. Use a carrier oil when needed or to case in the oils.

INTERNAL: Only use essential oils that are labeled for consumption from the Vitality line. You may add a drop or two into an empty capsule and top off with a carrier oil, use a drop under your tongue, add a drop to a glass or stainless steel water bottle, or add a drop to honey or another edible item.

Eucalyptus Leaves

Quality

Young Living's Seed to Seal®

"Young Living is proud to set the standard for essential oil purity and authenticity by carefully monitoring the production of our oils through our unique Seed to Seal process. From the time the seed is sourced until the oil is sealed in the bottle, we apply rigorous quality controls to ensure that you are receiving essential oils exactly the way nature intended."

STEP 1: **SEED** *Seeds are carefully selected by experts based on the previous year crop potency and effectiveness.*

STEP 2: **CULTIVATE** *Using only sustainable methods, our farming practices set the bar around the world.*

STEP 3: **DISTILL** *We are the largest innovator of oil distillation using several proprietary techniques.*

STEP 4: **TEST** *We test all oils using our internal labs, and 3rd party testing. Our standards are higher than international standards.*

STEP 5: **SEAL** *Each bottle is carefully packaged to ensure a perfect product shipped directly to you.*

www.seedtoseal.com

DERIVED FROM DR. COLE WOOLLEY

AUTHENTIC 100% PURE ~ SINGLE SPECIES

Authentic essential oils are 100% pure throughout the bottle. There are no added synthetics or other species of oils. They make up the small minority of all essential oils on the market.

MANIPULATED 100% PURE ~ MULT-SPECIES

Perfumers are often hired by essential oil companies to help make the final product smell more pleasing and less earthy. They will take away some of the heavier molecules or add very small amounts of another species to enhance the aroma.

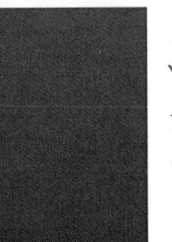

PERFUME PURE + SYNTHETIC

You will often see an essential oil labeled as "pure" when they are not. There is a percentage of pure essential oil and a percentage of synthetic to enhance the final aroma. These types of oils often cause headaches and do not have any therapeutic action.

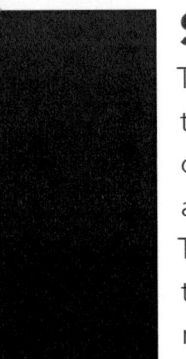

SYNTHETIC 100% SYNTHETIC

These "essential oils" are not essential oils at all. Because there are no labeling regulations on the term "essential oil," full synthetic oils are able to be labeled as pure and sold to unsuspecting consumers to increase profit. These often smell nothing like the original plant, but they can be very close, and that is why a consumer may not know they are synthetic and have possible severe negative reactions.

SOME THINGS TO CONSIDER

Personal care products contain some of the worst toxic chemicals. In a study by NIOSH, they tested 2,938 chemicals and found that 884 are toxic, 778 cause acute toxicity, 376 are skin and eye irritants, 314 may cause biological mutations, 218 may cause reproductive complications, and 146 may cause tumors. *Source: United States House of Representatives Report from the National Institute of Occupational Safety and Health (NIOSH), 1989.*

The EPA stated as of 1980 that there are 70,000 chemicals that have been introduced into our environment since 1950. It has been also stated by the US Congress that it is estimated there are 3,000 new chemicals introduced every year. *Source: EPA, "Your Guide to the Environmental Protection Agency," December 1980. "Technologies and Management Strategies for Hazardous Waste Control," March 1983 by the United States Congress, Office of Technology Assessment.*

There was an average of 150,000 emergency room treated injuries associated with household chemicals from 1997-2004. *Source: National Electronic Injury Surveillance System, 1997-2004 as stated in the 2007 Hazard Screening Report - Home and Family Maintenance Products – Household Chemicals by the Consumer Product Safety Commission.*

"Each year, 90,000 children are treated in emergency departments for unintentional poisonings. Nearly 40 die. 90% of poison incidents happen at home." *Source: The United States Consumer Product Safety Commission "Poison Prevention Poster," 2013.*

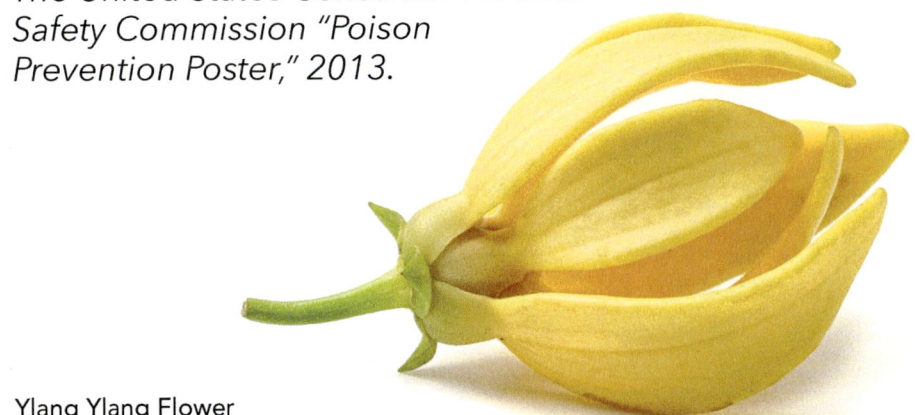

Ylang Ylang Flower

Lavender

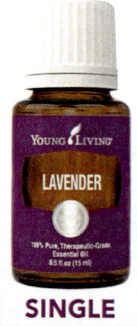

SINGLE

Lavender Fun Facts: Lavender is one of the most well-known and well-loved essential oils. It is commonly referred to as the "Swiss Army Knife" of oils. There is more synthetic Lavender on the market than the real thing, and Young Living's is the purest you can get. Young Living offers Lavender in the normal line as well as the Vitality line for consumption, but they are the exact same oil inside.

common uses

Internal with Vitality – Supports cardiovascular, immunity, respiratory, and nervous system.

Topical and Aromatic – Supports calming emotions, skin support, skin smoothing and soothing, seasonal support, hair strength, sleep support.

best practice

Internal with Vitality – Add 1-2 drops to a capsule for daily support.

Aromatic – Diffuse during the day for better focus. Diffuse at night for a more restful night's sleep.

Topical – Add a few drops to your daily face cream and serum. Add several drops to water in a spray bottle to mist over a pillow or to freshen a room.

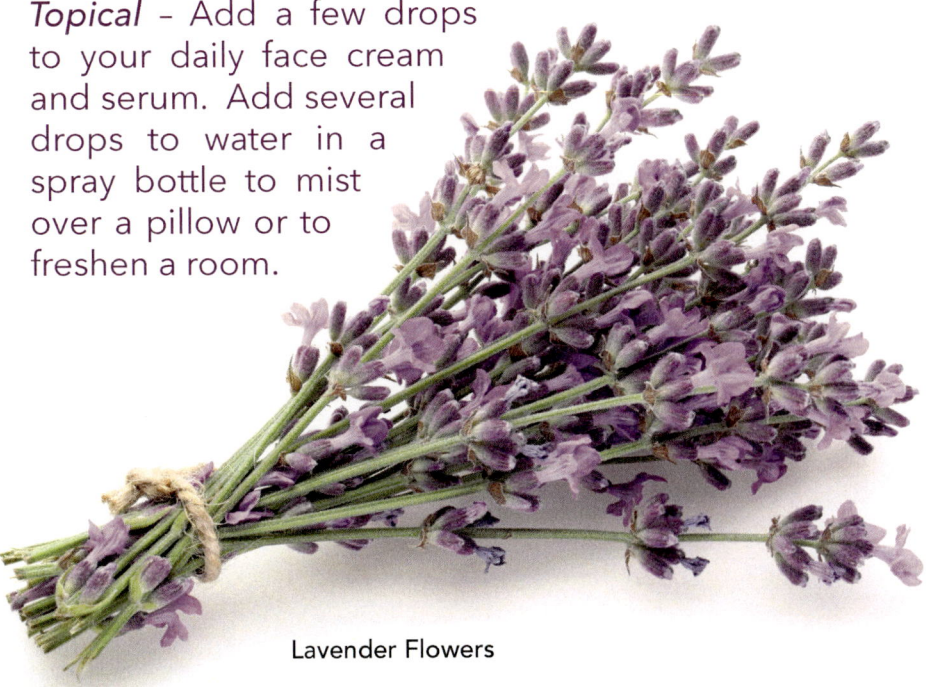

Lavender Flowers

Frankincense

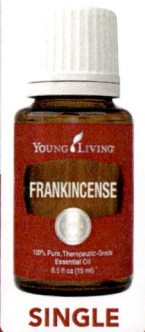

SINGLE

Frankincense Fun Facts:

Frankincense has been traded around the Middle East for over 5,000 years. The tree is cut, then the sap/resin that slowly oozes out of the tree and dries is collected and steam distilled. It is offered both in the normal and Vitality line through Young Living. They are the exact same oil inside, but the outside showcases different uses.

common uses

Internal with Vitality – Supports immunity and respiratory systems.

Topical and Aromatic – Calms mood, supports meditation, and enhances skin smoothing.

best practice

Internal with Vitality – Add a drop to a capsule for daily health support.

Topical – Apply a drop to the back of neck to support brain health and focus.

Aromatic – Diffuse for a relaxing and meditative experience.

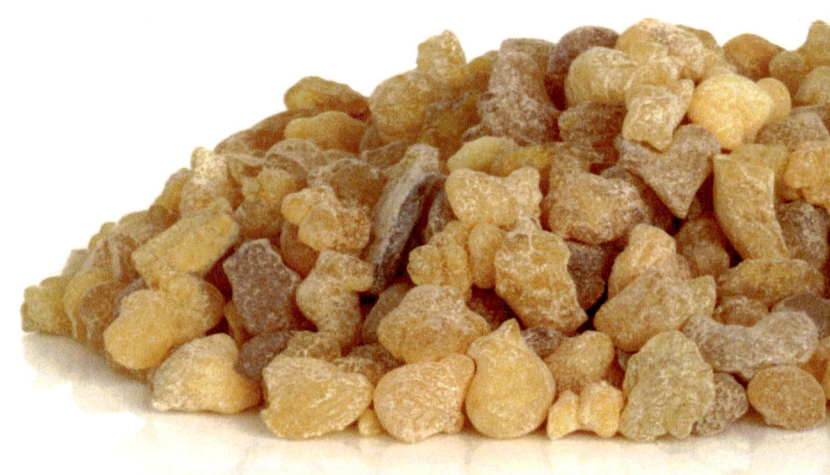

Frankincense Resin

Copaiba

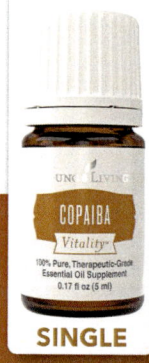

Copaiba Fun Facts: Copaiba, pronounced kō-pī-bah or kō-pī-ee-bah, is steam distilled from the oleoresin, which is a mixture of the essential oil and resin of the plant. It is excellent to help calm and soothe muscles and joints. It is offered both in the normal and Vitality line through Young Living. They are the exact same oil inside, but the outside showcases different uses.

common uses

Internal with Vitality – Supports cardiovascular, nervous, and respiratory systems.

Topical and Aromatic – Helpful to calm and focus the mind when diffused or applied topically. Helps to soothe muscle tension.

best practices

Internal with Vitality – Add a drop to a capsule to support healthful body systems.

Topical – Apply topically after strenuous exercise. Rub a drop on the back of the neck and temples to support calming cognitive support.

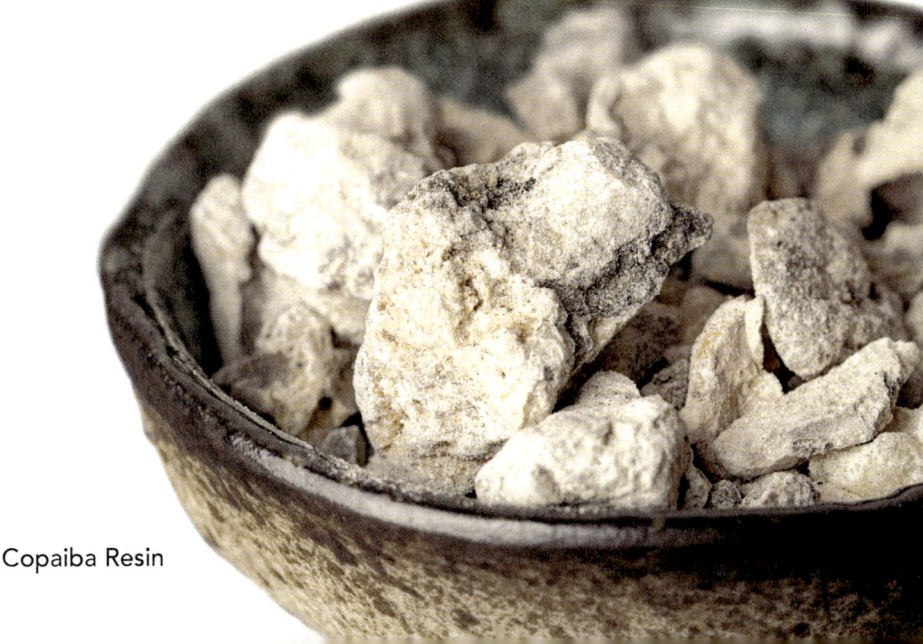

Copaiba Resin

Lemon

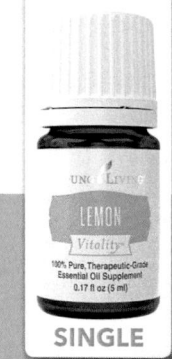

SINGLE

Lemon Fun Facts: It takes about 75 lemons to make one 15mL bottle of Lemon Essential Oil. It is cold pressed from the rind rather than steam distilled. It is so high in Monoterpenes, you can use it to clean the blackest grime off of surfaces with ease! Young Living offers Lemon in the normal line as well as the Vitality line for consumption, but they are the exact same oil inside the bottles.

common uses

Internal with Vitality – Supports immunity, digestive, respiratory; helps flush your renal system.

Topical and Aromatic – Helpful for uplifting moods; a grime dissolver and skin brightener.

best practices

Internal with Vitality – Place a drop in your glass or stainless steel water bottle for a refreshing boost to your cells and systems.

Topical – Apply to nail beds and rub in to support nail strength. Apply a drop to a greasy spot to dissolve.

Aromatic – Diffuse throughout the day for an uplifting, fresh, and clean aroma.

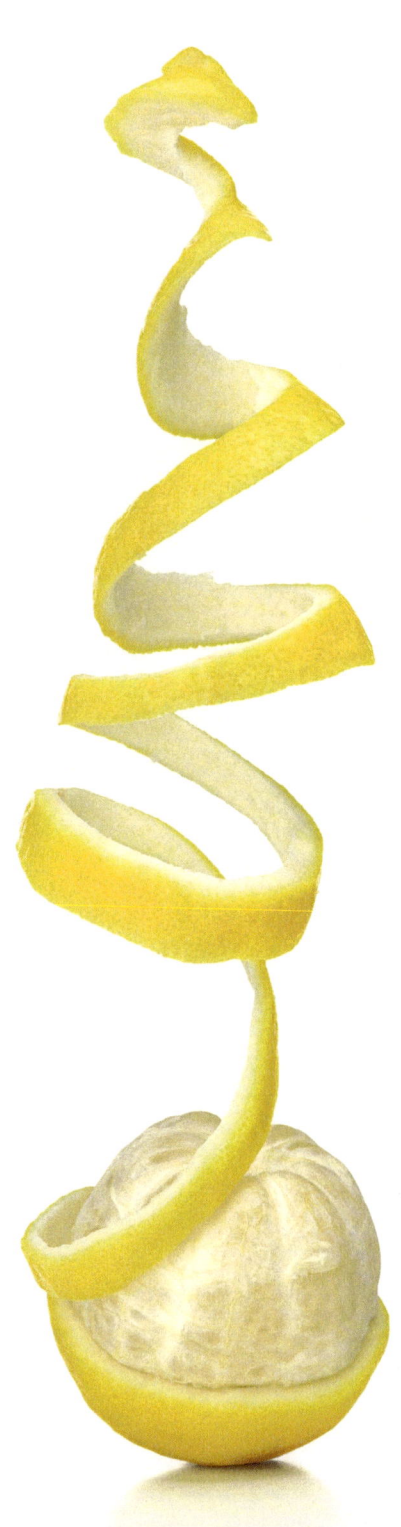

Lemon Fruit

Peppermint

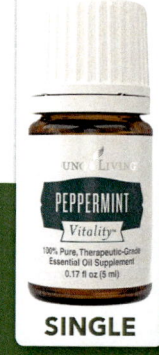

SINGLE

Peppermint Fun Facts: It takes about one pound of peppermint material to produce one 15mL bottle of Peppermint Essential Oil. It is a natural hybrid of Spearmint and Watermint. Peppermint is a driving oil that helps drive other oils in deeper and faster. It is offered both in the normal and Vitality line through Young Living. They are the exact same oil inside, but the outside showcases different uses.

common uses

Internal with Vitality – Circulatory and digestive support, airway support, cravings and appetite support.

Topical and Aromatic – Uplifting and energizing aroma, cooling sensation for topical use.

best practices

Internal with Vitality – Add a drop to your glass or stainless steel water bottle for a refreshing experience. Add a drop to a capsule topped off with carrier oil to help support healthy digestion and circulation.

Topical – Rub a drop on location with carrier oil after a strenuous workout. Apply a drop with carrier oil on temples and back of neck for a soothing cooling sensation.

Aromatic – Apply a drop on your hands and breathe in deeply to help uplift and open your airways.

Mint Leaves

Stress Away™

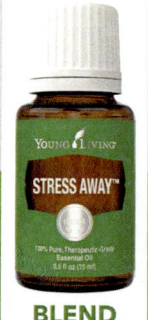

Stress Away™ Fun Facts: Stress Away is a customer favorite blend, and it's commonly joked that users would bathe in it if they could. It contains a small amount of Vanilla absolute, making it a favorite among kids and adults alike, with children often calling it their "vanilla ice cream oil." This blend contains 5 single oils: Copaiba, Lime, Cedarwood, Ocotea, and Lavender with a touch of Vanilla absolute.

common uses

Topical and Aromatic – Calming for emotions, helpful during times of stress, and great for better focus and mental clarity.

best practices

Topical – Rub a drop on the wrists and back of neck in the morning for a more focus-friendly day.

Aromatic – Add 6 drops to a cold water diffuser at night to calm the environment for a more restful sleep. Add 3-4 drops to a warm bath and enjoy a stress-free spa-like soak.

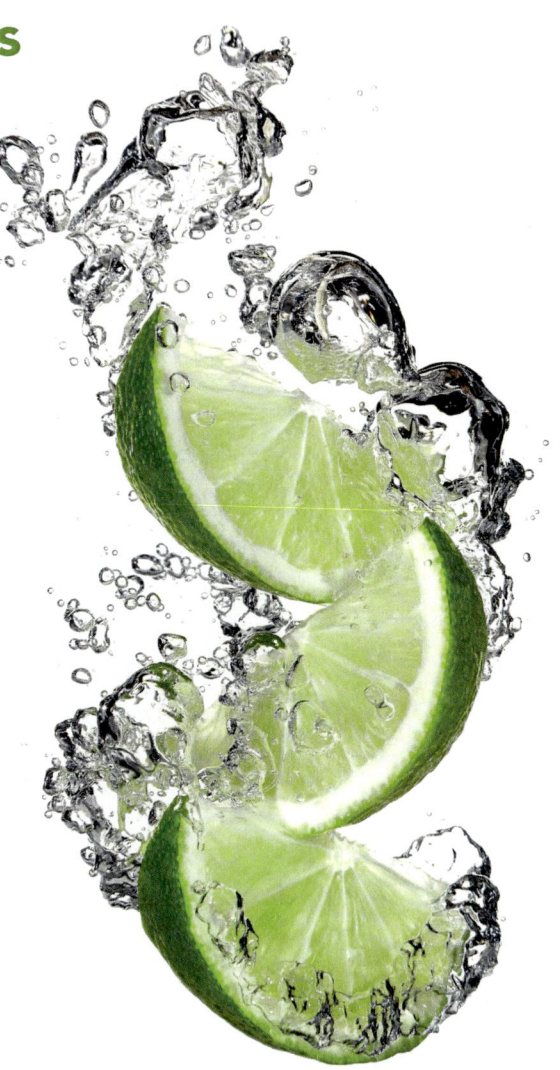

Lime Fruit

PanAway®

PanAway® Fun Facts:

When a person is in physical need of this blend, they usually smell it and love it! They say they could almost eat it (but don't do that since this oil is not for consumption!) PanAway has a childproof cap that indicates the oil is not for consumption. This blend contains 4 single oils: Wintergreen, Helichrysum, Clove, and Peppermint. Helichrysum is known for its regenerative properties.

common uses

Topical – Apply this oil with carrier oil for a refreshing after-workout experience or to help sooth tired muscles and feet after a long day.

best practices

Topical – This blend is best used topically. Apply on location liberally as needed. It is considered a hot oil, meaning it can feel biting, but has a cooling sensation, so it is best to use with a carrier oil.

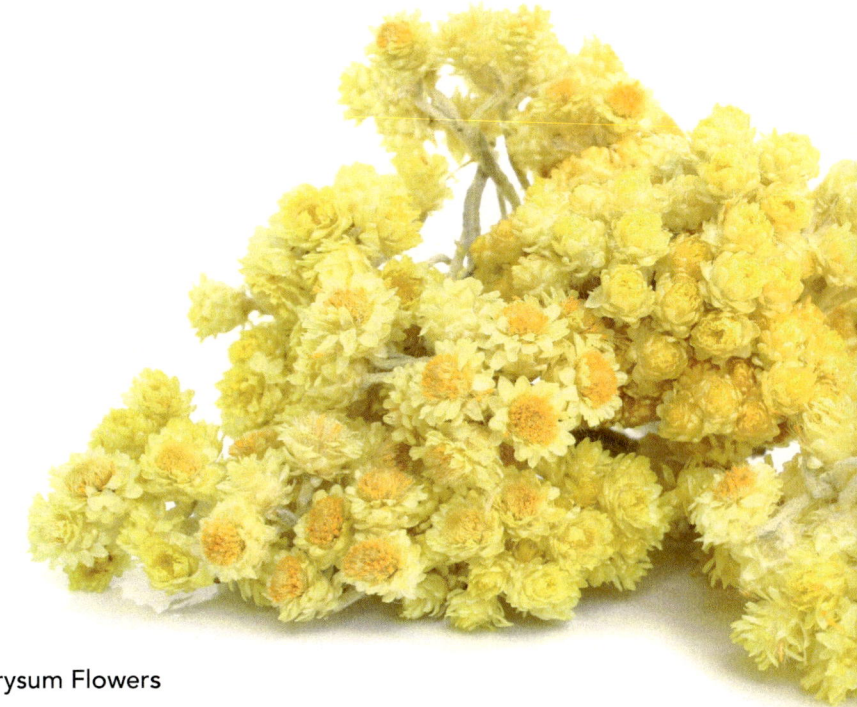

Helichrysum Flowers

Thieves®

Thieves® Fun Facts: The name "Thieves" comes from a legend about four thieves who rubbed on a similar blend before they robbed the dead and dying during the plague. It is offered both in the normal and Vitality line through Young Living. They are the exact same oil inside, but the outside showcases different uses. This blend contains 5 single oils: Clove, Lemon, Cinnamon Bark, Eucalyptus Radiata, and Rosemary.

common uses

Internal with Vitality – Immunity support.

Topical – Amazing fresh aroma, helps freshen the room.

best practices

Internal with Vitality – Add a drop to Ningxia Red® or add a drop to a capsule for a healthful morning routine.

Aromatic – Diffuse to keep air smelling clean and fresh.

Topical – Massage a drop to the bottom of the feet to support fresh-smelling feet.

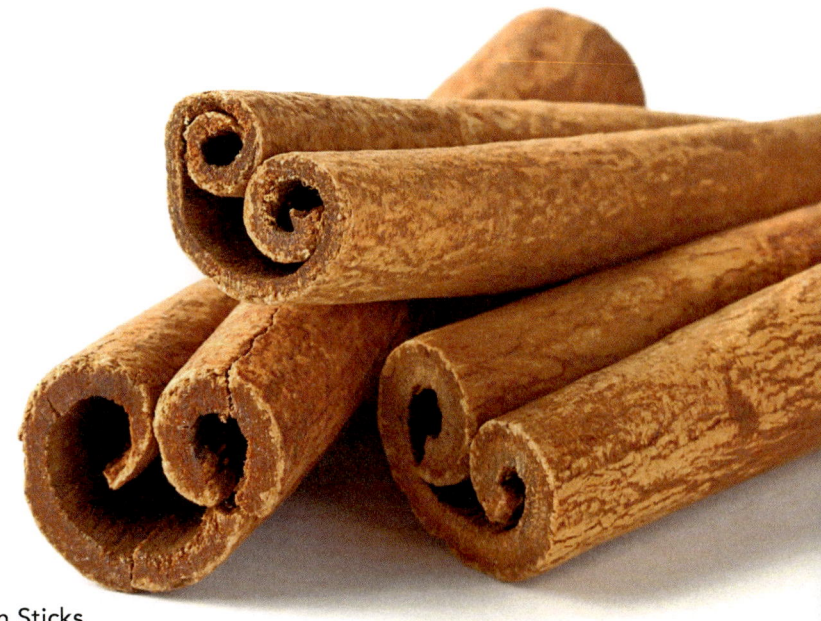

Cinnamon Sticks

RC™

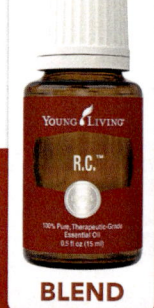

BLEND

RC™ Fun Facts: RC™ has gotten many nicknames over the years, such as Respiratory Care, Respiratory Comfort, and Respiratory Clearing. Eucalyptus Globulus is often noted to not be used on children; however, RC is formulated with littles in mind and is completely safe. This blend contains 10 single oils: Eucalyptus Globulus, Myrtle, Marjoram, Pine, Eucalyptus Radiata, Eucalyptus Citriodora, Lavender, Cypress, Black Spruce, and Peppermint.

common uses

Topical and Aromatic – Calming and flushing for healthy airways.

best practices

Aromatic – Diffuse for a calming and relaxing environment.

Topical – Rub a drop on the chest and the back to encourage respiratory clearing.

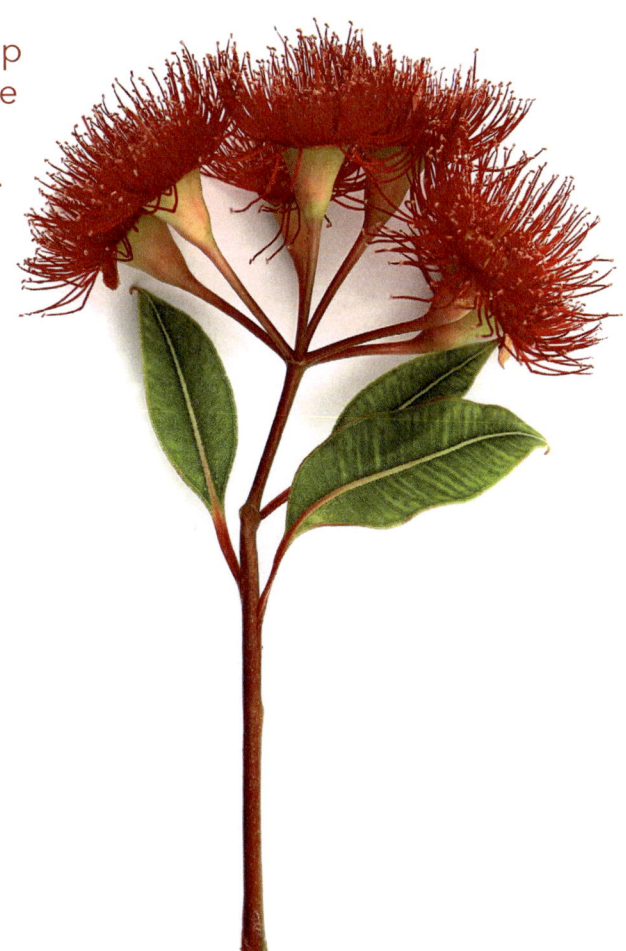

Red Eucalyptus Flowers

DiGize™

DiGize™ Fun Facts: A life-saver for many people, DiGize™ has been known to help calm digestion just by holding the bottle! Many people do not leave home without it. It is offered both in the normal and Vitality line through Young Living. They are the exact same oil inside, but the outside showcases different uses. This blend contains 8 single oils: Tarragon, Ginger, Peppermint, Juniper, Fennel, Lemongrass, Anise, and Patchouli.

common uses

Internal with Vitality – Digestive support and intestinal support.

Topical – Calming and cleansing.

best practices

Internal with Vitality – Add a drop under the tongue to support systems. Add 2 drops to a capsule with carrier oil to support digestion.

Aromatic – Diffuse for a fresh aroma.

Topical – Rub a drop on the abdomen clockwise to help promote healthy movement and counter-clockwise to slow down movement.

Ginger Root

Purification®

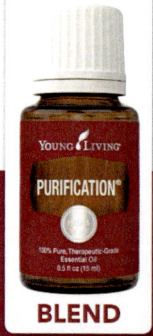

BLEND

Purification® Fun Facts:

Purification® is the oil most commonly used to freshen stinky feet. One drop on the bottom of the feet in the morning gets the job done. It is also a mom favorite for their school-age kids to help keep critters away. It has a fresh, Lemongrass aroma that is wonderfully neutralizing. This blend contains 6 single oils: Citronella, Rosemary, Lemongrass, Tea Tree, Lavandin, and Myrtle.

common uses

Aromatic – Diffuse to freshen the room.

Topical – General body odor support.

best practices

Aromatic – Diffuse to neutralize odors in a room. Put one drop on a cotton ball and place in car to freshen the air. Apply a couple drops to paint before applying to the walls for a fresher experience.

Topical – Apply a drop to the bottom of the feet every morning on kids to help keep critters away and to help support fresh-smelling feet.

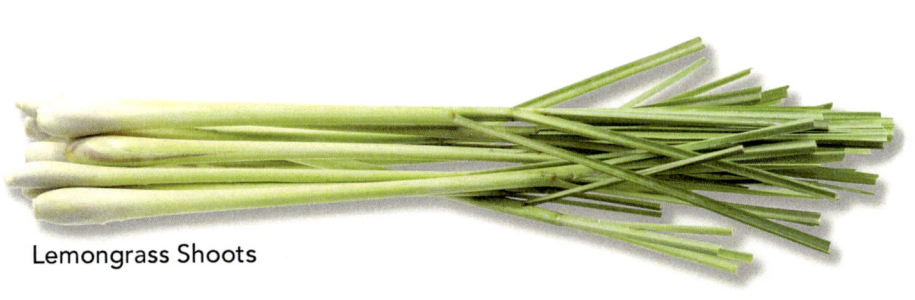

Lemongrass Shoots

Ningxia Red®

Ningxia Red® is a whole body supplement for a more healthful life experience. The wolfberry, also known as the goji berry, is touted for having high antioxidant properties. A daily shot helps support better energy and normal cellular function, as well as whole-body health and wellness. Four ounces of Ningxia Red® equals one serving of fruit; however, one ounce has the antioxidant equivalent to eating 4lbs of carrots or 8 whole oranges!

common uses
Drink one ounce daily to support health.

best practices
In the morning, drink one ounce of Ningxia Red® alone or mix it up and add one drop of Thieves Vitality™ or Frankincense Vitality™. In the afternoon, drink one ounce and add one drop of Tangerine Vitality™ or Longevity Vitality™ or any oil from the Vitality™ line.

is it safe?
Ningxia Red® is safe for all people from solid-food eating children to adults. Pregnant and nursing women should also consider using it as part of their daily regimen.

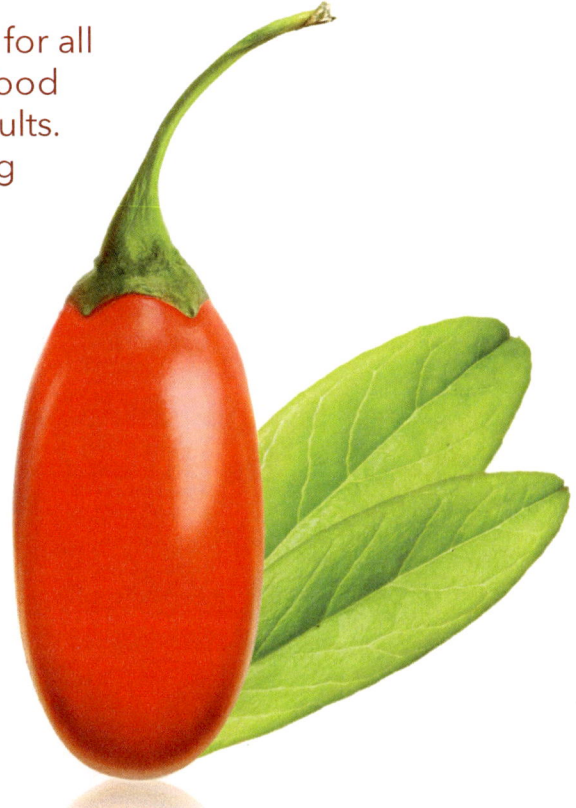

Goji Berry aka Wolfberry

Diffusers

Cold-water diffusers are essential to any family that wants to promote a more healthful environment.

BENEFITS OF DIFFUSING

Supports more restful sleep.

Supports better daytime focus.

Promotes healthy air quality.

Helps force dust to the floor.

Creates a healthy ionized room.

Promotes an uplifting environment.

Helps neutralize odors.

Safer alternative to candles.

Helps to elevate moods.

Promotes better energy.

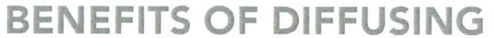

YOUNG LIVING

The Aria™

exploring the diffusers

The Aria™ *Ultrasonic Diffuser* – Gorgeous glass dome with a solid American maple wood base, this diffuser comes complete with multiple settings from 1-8 hours, a range of LED color options, plus it plays relaxing spa-inspired music or you may plug in your own personal music device. It's an ultrasonic atomizer and humidifier all in one.

The Rainstone™ *Diffuser* – This stylish black high-end clay base ultrasonic atomizer and humidifying diffuser comes with multiple settings including timer from 1-8 hours, LED control with various color options, as well as the ability to turn on or off the ionizer.

The Dewdrop™ *Diffuser* – This workhorse diffuser is also a family favorite. It is the only silent diffuser and features 4 hours of run-time with automatic shut-off. It is an ultrasonic atomizer and humidifier all in one.

The Home Diffuser – The home diffuser, with a rose-inspired shape, is an ultrasonic atomizer and humidifier all-in-one easy-to-use product. It features 4 hours of run-time or a 30 second burst for up to 8 hours.

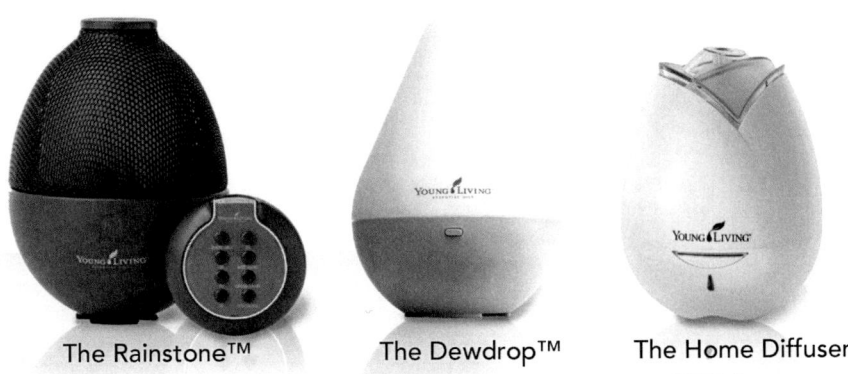

The Rainstone™   The Dewdrop™   The Home Diffuser

the more you know

There are 85-100 drops per 5mL bottle.

There are 250-300 drops per 15mL bottle.

"Hot" means the oil may feel warm or hot.

"Neat" means you may apply without a carrier oil.

Carrier oils, like Grapeseed, dilute an essential oil.

If essential oils get in your eye, rinse with rice milk.

Don't apply citrus oils to the skin if going in the sun.

Always dilute with carrier oil for those under age 12.

If you experience an uncomfortable response, add carrier oil or discontinue use.

The statements in this booklet are for educational purposes only. They are not intended to diagnose, treat, or cure any disease or illness.

how to order...

Purity is key when choosing the right essential oil company. The right person to assist you on your journey is also important. My goal is to help you learn the right way to use your essential oils, and also share more ways to add health and wellness to your family and home. There are several ways you can get started. Ask me how to become a wholesale member with Young Living Essential Oils.

BENEFITS OF MEMBERSHIP

- 24% off retail prices

- Discount of over 50% off the retail price of the Premium Starter Kit.

- No additional fees, your kit purchase is your membership fee.

- No minimum monthly orders.

- Order what you want, when you want.

- Access to Essential Rewards to get up to an additional 25% back on your monthly order.

- Access to a group of health-conscious people who are on the same path!

Blue Tansy

Made in the USA
Middletown, DE
20 July 2017

HEALTH & FITNESS / Aromatherapy
LIST PRICE: $7.99

This simple little manual is a perfect addition to your Premium Starter Kit with Young Living Essential Oils. It helps you unpack each item with tips and usage ideas to get you started. It's an Essential Oil 101 class wrapped up in a pretty, simple, and fun little book.

Live well.

www.31oils.com

ISBN 9781546752905

90000

9 781546 752905

Righteousness
By
Faith

Transcription

of

Larry
Wilson